I0774528

EASY CHAIR YOGA ROUTINE FOR SENIORS

A comprehensive guide to unlocking vitality and discovering the art of wellness that includes mind-blowing methods for strong joints and gentle sitting exercises for healthy aging.

Shirlene Roberson

Copyright @ 2024 by Shirlene Roberson

All rights reserved

No part of this book may be used or
reproduced in any form whatsoever
without written permission except in the
case of brief quotations in critical articles
or reviews.

Table of Contents

INTRODUCTION 1

Embracing Senior Chair Yoga 1

Recognizing the Advantages of Chair Yoga for Elderly People...1

Safety Procedures and Guidelines....................2

A Restorative Story Using Chair Yoga 3

CHAPTER 1...5

Accepting Chair Yoga's Foundations 5

Establishing a Comfortable Space 5

Selecting the Correct Chair 6

Appropriate Breathing Methods.......................6

CHAPTER 2...9

Warm-up Pose for Sitting: Taking Care of Your Body with Calm Motions.....................................9

Shoulder and Neck Rolls: 9

Mild Arm Stretches 11

Toe Taps and Ankle Circles 12

CHAPTER 3 15

Core Stabilization Practices: Establishing Center-Based Stability and Vitality 15

Cat-Cow Stretch in Sitting 15

Twist for Spinal Mobility While Seated 16

Contractions of the Abdomen for Core Stability .. 17

CHAPTER 4 19

Joint Flexibility Exercises: Improving Senior Mobility 19

Ankle and Wrist Flexes 19

Lifting and extending the knee 20

Mobility-Boosting Hip Openers 21

CHAPTER 5 23

Posture and Balance Exercises: Promoting Stability and Proper Alignment in Seniors 23

Mountain Pose while Sitting 23

Leg Extensions for Balance 24

Sitting Spinal Alignment 25

CHAPTER 6..27

Chair Yoga as a Means of Relaxation and Stress Reduction...27

Meditation and Mindful Breathing.................27

Guided Relaxation Methods...........................28

Chair Yoga Nidra for Profound Relaxation.......29

CHAPTER 7..31

Daily Chair Yoga Practices: Energize, Relax, and Unwind..31

Morning Energizer Routine:...........................31

1.   Seated Cat-Cow Stretch...............................31

2.   Leg Extensions for Balance.......................32

3.   Mountain Pose: Sit with your feet flat and your spine straight...32

Afternoon Relaxation Session 33

Wind-down Poses for Bedtime 35

CHAPTER 8..37

Customizing Yoga Positions to Meet Everybody's Needs 37

Adapting Pose to Various Abilities 37

Chair Yoga for Those with Limited Mobility 39

Answering Frequently Asked Questions and Providing Clarity and Comfort in Yoga Practice40

CHAPTER 9..43

A Holistic Approach to Wellness: Including Chair Yoga in Daily Life 43

Practical tips to help improve your routine.....45

CONCLUSION 47

Embrace wellness through chair yoga. 47

Honoring Chair Yoga's Benefits for Seniors 47

Motivation to Maintain Physical Activity and Good Health 48

Bonus...51

Mental wellness through mindful moments 51

INTRODUCTION

Embracing Senior Chair Yoga

It's easy to forget how important it is to preserve our physical and mental well-being in the midst of the daily grind, particularly as we become older. This introduction seeks to shed light on the profoundly positive effects of chair yoga on seniors' general health and energy, while also providing a compelling case study for its use.

Recognizing the Advantages of Chair Yoga for Elderly People

Chair yoga is designed with the special requirements of older citizens in mind, offering a gentle and approachable introduction to the practice of yoga. The benefits of chair yoga are many and deep, ranging from improving balance and flexibility to supporting joint health and lowering stress. We'll explore a carefully chosen range of yoga positions and practices on the pages that follow, all aimed at empowering seniors to take charge of their path toward better health.

Safety Procedures and Guidelines

It's important to put safety first before starting any exercise regimen. Readers who read this part will be equipped with the necessary instructions to ensure a safe and comfortable chair yoga practice. We stress the need of customizing the practice to each person's ability, from appropriate body alignment to progressive advancement.

Introducing Mary, a lively senior whose days were formerly marred by bothersome knee problems and nagging bodily aches. Mary became frustrated with the restrictions these illnesses placed on her day-to-day activities and learned about the therapeutic benefits of chair yoga.

Mary felt a power and relief she hadn't felt in years as she embraced the soft stances and deliberate movements. Her refuge became the yoga practice, and the chair served as her support. Mary's physical aches gradually disappeared with regular exercise, and her reticent knees started to move with unexpected freedom. Chair yoga gave her a sense of strength and gave new life and pleasure to her senior years.

Mary's tale demonstrates both the human spirit's tenacity and the transformational power of chair yoga for older citizens. It reminds us that it's never too late to start along the path to better health and wellbeing, which should inspire all readers. Let Mary's journey serve as a beacon of hope as we delve into the numerous chair yoga techniques that lie ahead, demonstrating the transformative power of mindful movement for older citizens.

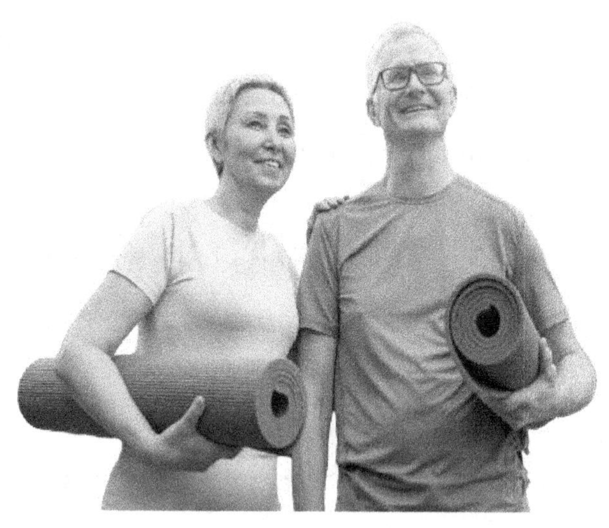

CHAPTER 1

Accepting Chair Yoga's Foundations

Starting a chair yoga practice entails setting up the foundation for a cozy and fulfilling routine. We explore the fundamental components that create the conditions for a successful and happy experience in this part.

Establishing a Comfortable Space

The secret to reaping the full benefits of chair yoga is to create a setting that is favorable. Choose an area that is peaceful, well-lit, and unobstructed so that you may walk about easily. Place your chair such that it is stable in all positions and that it doesn't slide. To improve the whole experience, add calming aspects to the environment, such as gentle lighting or relaxing music.

Selecting the Correct Chair

Your comfort and support throughout the practice are greatly influenced by the chair you choose. Select a robust chair with a straight back and a flat, solid seat. When doing standing poses, armrests may give extra support, and keeping your feet comfortably on the floor encourages good alignment. Finding a chair that supports a stable and well-balanced base for your yoga practice is the aim.

Appropriate Breathing Methods

Breath is the living force that gives your practice vigor. Learning the correct breathing techniques is essential for concentration and relaxation in chair yoga. To begin, practice breathing awareness by inhaling deeply and slowly through your nose, then softly expelling through your mouth. Sync each position with a conscious breathing cycle to create a seamless integration of breath and movement. In addition to increasing the efficiency of the yoga postures, the focus on conscious breathing fosters attention and tranquility.

Recall that your path is distinct as you go through these fundamental elements of chair yoga. You create the foundation for a gratifying and transforming practice by arranging your surroundings comfortably, selecting the ideal chair, and adopting the perfect breathing methods. Chair yoga's strength comes from its attentive integration of breath and movement, which not only improves physical postures but also promotes a well-rounded approach to wellbeing.

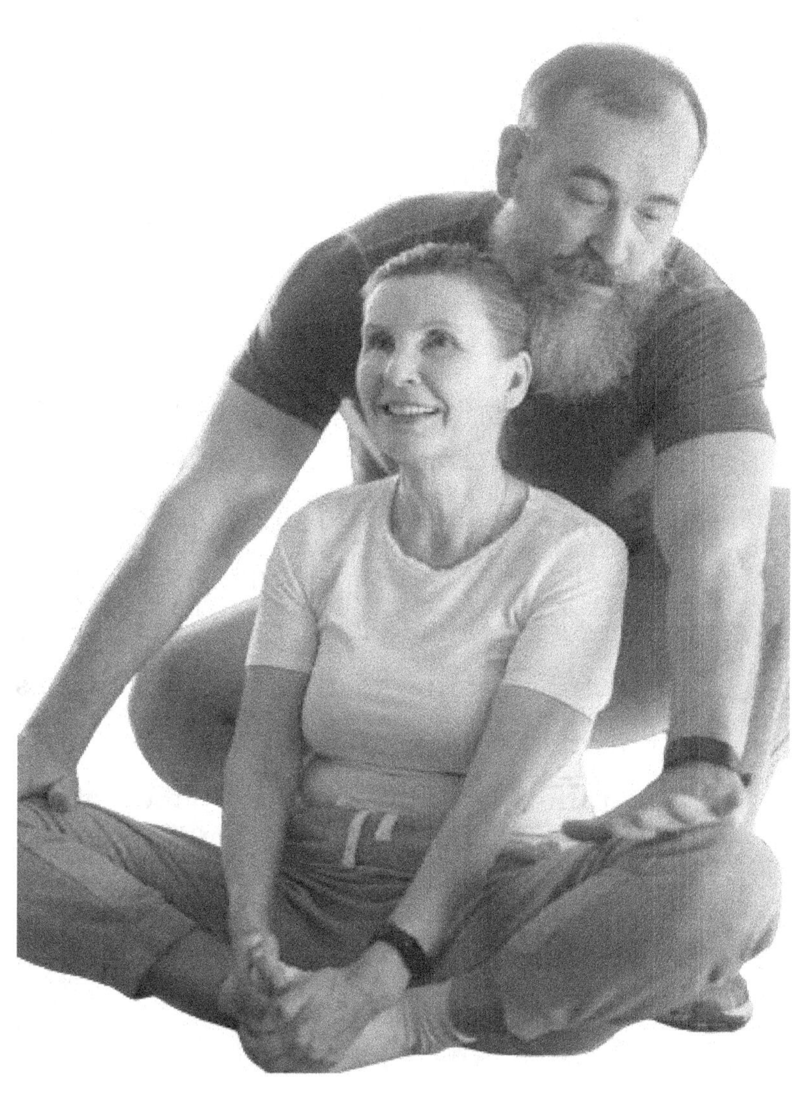

CHAPTER 2

Warm-up Pose for Sitting: Taking Care of Your Body with Calm Motions

It's important to include sitting warm-up poses into your chair yoga practice to prime your body for the more dynamic stretches that lie ahead. These mild motions improve blood flow and suppleness, laying the groundwork for a more relaxed and productive practice.

Shoulder and Neck Rolls:

- Start by maintaining a straight spine and a comfortable position on your chair.
- Take a deep breath in, and then release it while slowly lowering your chin to your chest and rotating your neck in a clockwise direction.

- Take a breath as you raise your head back to the center, and release it as you rotate your neck counterclockwise.
- Repeat this routine a few times, letting your shoulders and neck relax with the light motions.

Tip: Proceed cautiously and gently to provide a strain-free, smooth action. This relieves stiffness and enhances neck flexibility.

Health Benefits: Shoulder and neck rolls reduce stress, increase cervical spine flexibility, and promote circulation. Additionally, by relieving stiffness, these motions encourage relaxation and relieve tension that is often stored in the shoulders and neck.

Mild Arm Stretches

- You start by sitting upright is the first step. As you raise your arms over your head, take a breath and exhale.
- Then, slowly tilt your head to one side and feel the stretch go through your arm and along your side.
- Return your breath to the center, and then release it as you tilt to the other side.
- Continue stretching from side to side, progressively increasing the range of motion.
- These exercises increase upper body flexibility and relieve stress in the shoulders and sides. Use caution while moving, and only extend as far as it feels comfortable for you. Feeling a little stretch is the aim; don't try to force your body into pain.

Health Benefits: Light arm stretches improve upper back, shoulder, and arm flexibility. They increase circulation and range of motion, which lowers the chance of stiffness and improves mobility throughout the upper body.

Toe Taps and Ankle Circles

- First place your feet flat on the floor while sitting.
- Elevate one foot a little and start gently rotating your ankle in a clockwise manner.
- Change to rotating in a counterclockwise direction after a few turns.
- Carry out the same action with the other foot. To do a toe tap, raise one foot and tap the bottom of it, then go to the other foot.

These exercises improve ankle flexibility, increase circulation, and warm up the lower body.

Tip: Take your time and walk carefully while focusing on your ankle and foot feelings. Seniors who want to preserve or enhance their lower extremity mobility will especially benefit from this.

Health Benefits: Ankle circles help to increase the flexibility and mobility of joints, which lowers the chance of pain and stiffness. Toe tapping helps to enhance circulation and balance by activating the muscles in the lower legs and strengthening the feet.

Including these sitting warm-up positions in your chair yoga practice will guarantee that your body is sufficiently warmed up for the postures that follow. Let these soft motions awaken and energize your body in a safe, thoughtful way as you take the time to connect with your breath and enjoy their delicate nature.

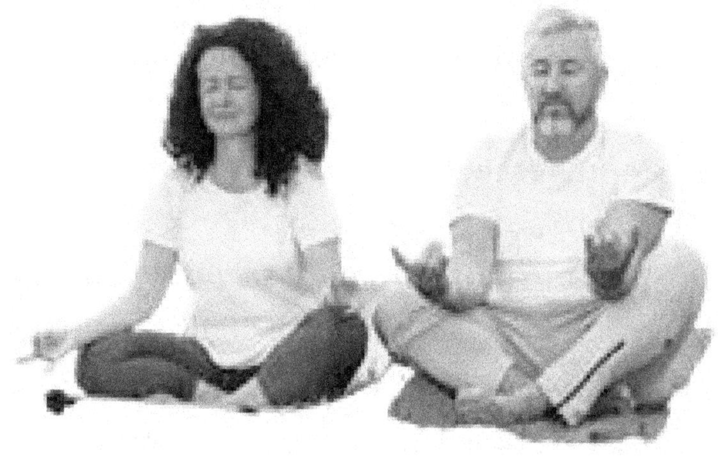

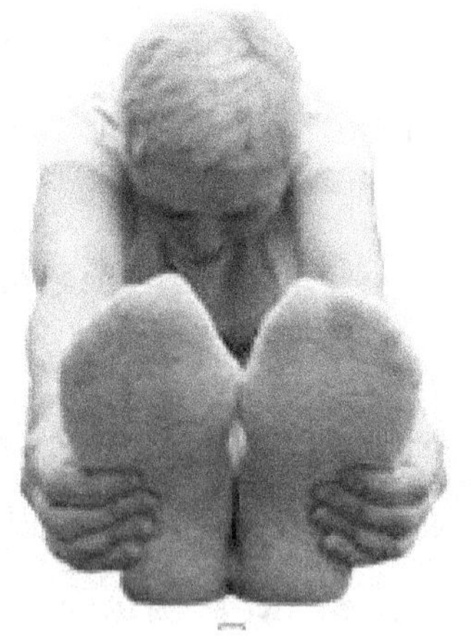

CHAPTER 3

Core Stabilization Practices: Establishing Center-Based Stability and Vitality

For general stability and wellbeing, it is essential to engage and develop the core. The purpose of the following chair yoga postures is to strengthen the muscles of the core, improve spinal mobility, and develop a strong center.

Cat-Cow Stretch in Sitting

- Sit with your back straight and your hands on your knees to start.
- Taking a deep breath, raise your chest and push your pelvis forward to form the cow pose.

- Pull your chin to your chest and release the breath as you circle your spine (Cat Pose).
- Continue the flowing motion while synchronizing your breathing with your spine's curving and arching.

Health Benefits: The seated cat-cow stretch strengthens the back muscles, opens up the spine, and works the core. This dynamic movement improves the spinal column's overall range of motion, reducing stiffness and encouraging a flexible, healthy back.

Twist for Spinal Mobility While Seated

- Sit with your feet flat on the ground and a tall spine.
- Breathe in as you extend your back and out as you rotate to the side, supporting one hand on the chair's back and the other on the knee across from you.

- Feel the stretch throughout your spine as you hold the twist for a few breaths. Continue on the other side.

Health Benefits: The Seated Twist improves spinal flexibility, stretches the back muscles, and promotes better digestion. Moreover, twisting postures aid in detoxifying by relieving stress and assisting the body in getting rid of waste.

Contractions of the Abdomen for Core Stability

- Take a comfortable seat and put your hands on your thighs.
- Take a deep breath and stretch your abdomen.
- When you completely exhale, contract your abdominal muscles and pull your navel inside toward your spine.
- Before releasing, hold the contraction for a little while.

Health Benefits: By fortifying the core muscles, abdominal contractions help to improve posture and stabilize the spine. Additionally, this practice improves respiratory capacity, aids in improved digestion, and raises general core awareness.

To develop a strong and steady center, include these chair yoga postures that strengthen the core. As your core strength becomes stronger over time, progressively increase the intensity of each exercise while maintaining mindfulness of your breathing.

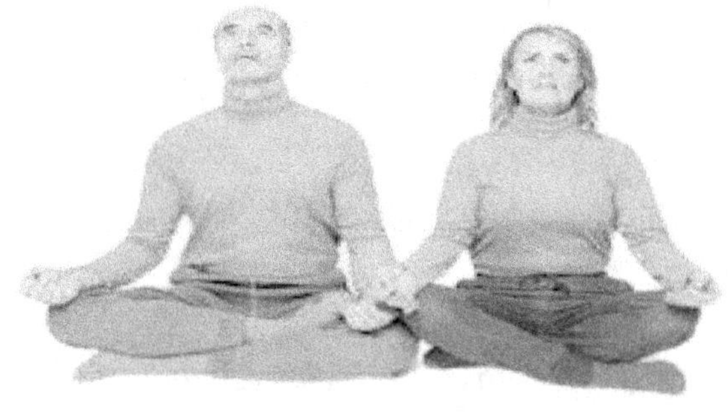

CHAPTER 4

Joint Flexibility Exercises: Improving Senior Mobility

Seniors, picture a sitting exercise that elegantly works on joint flexibility, opening doors to a world of ease and mobility. The goal of these exercises is to improve your overall joint health by strengthening the flexibility of your knees, hips, ankles, and wrists.

<u>Ankle and Wrist Flexes</u>

- Start by raising your arms in front of you with your palms pointing downward for wrist flexes. Start by flexing your wrists by bringing them up and down slowly. Imagine using your fingers to make circles in the air.
- Exert one leg and rotate your ankle in both clockwise and

counterclockwise directions to do ankle flexes. On the opposite leg, repeat.

Health Benefits: Flexing your wrists improves dexterity and relieves stiffness, which are important for everyday duties. Ankle flexes are especially helpful for those who lead sedentary lives since they increase mobility, decrease edema, and improve circulation.

Lifting and extending the knee

- (Knee Lifts): Lift one knee toward your chest while sitting. Hold the position for a little while before lowering it. Switch between the legs.
- (Knee Extensions): Bend the foot in your direction after extending one leg forward. Repeat on the opposite leg,

Health Benefits: The range of motion and flexibility of the knee joints are improved with knee lifts and extensions. Enhancing leg strength is another benefit of these workouts, which is important for preserving equilibrium and avoiding falls.

Mobility-Boosting Hip Openers

- Sit with your feet flat on the ground and your back straight.
- Bring the soles of your feet together and extend your knees to the sides.
- Gently push your knees toward the floor while holding onto your ankles.

Health Benefits: Hip openers release tightness in the lower back and hips. Seniors who have improved hip mobility will have a wider range of motion, which will make sitting and walking more pleasant.

Imagine your body's joints gently opening up as you do these joint flexibility exercises, promoting greater range of motion. Accept these movements as a way to improve general health, relieve stiffness, and support joint health. These exercises address the special requirements of seniors, cultivating joint flexibility and fostering a feeling of vitality, whether your goal is to improve everyday functioning or you're just looking for a more flexible and pleasant lifestyle.

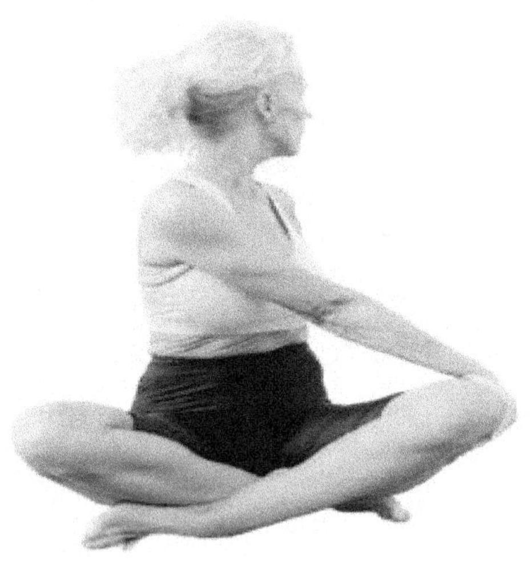

CHAPTER 5

Posture and Balance Exercises: Promoting Stability and Proper Alignment in Seniors

Try incorporating these chair yoga postures into your practice to improve posture, balance, and stability in general. Let's examine the detailed directions for every activity and the health advantages they provide.

<u>*Mountain Pose while Sitting*</u>:

- Take a comfortable seat with your feet flat on the ground. Lengthen your spine and use your sit bones to ground yourself.
- Raise your arms over your head, reaching upward with your palms facing each other.

- Take a deep breath and see yourself firmly planted like a mountain.

Health Benefits: By enhancing spinal alignment, seated mountain pose helps to enhance posture. It improves general stability, strengthens the back, and works the core muscles. Additionally, this stance promotes attention and a grounded feeling of being.

Leg Extensions for Balance

- Sit with both feet flat on the ground and a straight back.
- Straighten out one leg in front of you while maintaining its parallel to the floor.
- Using your core to maintain stability, hold for a few breaths.
- Repeat on the opposite side after lowering the leg.

Health Benefits: The muscles involved in balance are strengthened and challenged by leg extensions. Enhancing stability and coordination via exercise is essential in avoiding falls. It also strengthens the quadriceps and increases hip joint suppleness.

Sitting Spinal Alignment

- Take a comfortable seat with your feet flat on the ground. Breathe in as you extend your back and see your vertebrae piling one on top of the other.
- Breathe out while slowly moving your shoulders back and down. Retain an impartial and level-headed stance.

Health Benefits: By promoting a straight and extended spine, seated spinal alignment helps people maintain good posture. It lessens the chance of pain and discomfort by releasing tension in the shoulders and back. Better respiration and an enhanced sense of general wellbeing are correlated with improved spinal alignment.

While doing these balancing and posture postures, concentrate on how breath, movement, and attentive awareness are integrated. Regular engagement with these exercises fosters an internal feeling of balance in addition to improving physical alignment and stability. These chair yoga positions address the special requirements of seniors, promoting a harmonious connection between body and mind, whether your goal is to improve posture, avoid falls, or just live a more centered and grounded life.

CHAPTER 6

Chair Yoga as a Means of Relaxation and Stress Reduction

Try these peaceful chair yoga poses as part of your regimen to help you de-stress, induce deep relaxation, and unwind. Let's examine the detailed directions for every activity and the health advantages they provide.

Meditation and Mindful Breathing

- Take a comfortable seat, sit up straight, and place your hands on your lap.
- Shut your eyes and concentrate on your breathing.
- Take a deep breath through your nose and feel your belly and chest expand.

- Release tension by taking a slow, deep breath out of your lips. Let rid of outside distractions and concentrate on each breath.

Health Benefits: By encouraging relaxation and developing present-moment awareness, mindful breathing and meditation help lower stress. This exercise increases emotional stability, promotes inner peace, and sharpens mental focus.

Guided Relaxation Methods

- Take a seat in a comfortable posture. Shut your eyes and focus your attention on various body areas.
- Tension and release should be applied to every muscle group, working your way up to the head from your toes.

- Visualize yourself being swept away by a calm wave.

Health Benefits: Physical strain and emotional stress are reduced by guided relaxation methods. This technique generates a profound sensation of peace and aids in the release of accumulated stress by methodically relaxing the body, which enhances general well-being.

Chair Yoga Nidra for Profound Relaxation

- ***To practice:*** Take a comfortable seat or lie down on your chair. Shut your eyes and follow the script as it guides you to focus on breath, different sensations, and visions.
- Let your body and mind to sink into a deeply relaxed state, akin to a conscious slumber.

Health Benefits: Chair Yoga Nidra creates a profoundly relaxed state that lowers stress and enhances mental and emotional health. Improved mood, a feeling of inner serenity, and better sleep quality have all been linked to this exercise.

As you do these relaxation and stress-reduction exercises, settle into a peaceful space and give yourself permission to be present. Adding these activities to your regimen on a regular basis will help you live a calmer, more balanced lifestyle. Chair yoga offers seniors and people of all ages a moderate route to relaxation and stress reduction, whether they are looking for respite from everyday worries or just want to develop a stronger feeling of serenity.

CHAPTER 7

Daily Chair Yoga Practices: Energize, Relax, and Unwind

These chair yoga poses may be easily incorporated into your daily routine to help you find calm before bed, relax in the afternoon, and have a good start to your mornings. Here is a breakdown of each routine's steps:

<u>Morning Energizer Routine:</u>

1. ***Seated Cat-Cow Stretch***

    - Sit upright in your chair with your hands on your knees. This is the morning energy routine.
    - Take a breath, rising your chest and arching your back (Cat).

- Let out a breath, tucking your chin and rounding your spine (Cow).

- Synchronize movement with breathing and repeat for one to two minutes.

2. Leg Extensions for Balance

- Sit with both feet flat and your back straight.

- Raise one leg and straighten it while using your core.

- Switch legs after a few breaths of holding.

- Perform 10–12 repetitions for each leg.

3. Mountain Pose: Sit with your feet flat and your spine straight.

- Take a breath and raise your arms overhead, palms facing each other.

- Breathe deeply while you engage your core and hold for one to two minutes.
- Visualize yourself as a mountain with roots.

Health Benefits: The Morning Energizer Routine encourages flexibility, circulation, and mental clarity. It gives you a healthy start to the day and gets your body and mind ready for what is ahead.

<u>*Afternoon Relaxation Session*</u>

1) **Assisted Relaxation Methods**
   - Choose a chair that is comfortable for you.
   - Shut your eyes, tighten and relax every muscle in your body.
   - Visualize a wave of calmness enveloping you.

- Take five to ten minutes to methodically unwind your body.

2) ***Twist While Seated for Spinal Mobility***

- Sit upright, take a deep breath, and rotate your torso to one side.

- Feel the stretch while holding onto the chair for support.

- Let out and tighten the twist. For 30 seconds, hold.

- Proceed to the other side.

3) ***Meditation and Mindful Breathing***

- Take a comfortable seat and shut your eyes.

- Take a deep breath through your nose and release it through your lips.

- Let go of thoughts and concentrate on your breathing.

- For five to ten minutes, practice.

Health Benefits: The afternoon relaxation session eases stress and promotes mental clarity by releasing tension that has built up over the day. It creates a peaceful environment for the rest of the day.

Wind-down Poses for Bedtime

1. ***Chair Yoga Nidra for Profound Relaxation***
   - Take a comfortable seat or lie back in your chair.
   - Shut your eyes and adhere to the suggested script.
   - Permit yourself to sink into a profound state of relaxation.
   - Before going to bed, practice for ten to fifteen minutes.
2. ***Seated Spinal Alignment***
   - Sit with your feet flat and your spine straight.

- Take a breath, extend your spine, release it, and straighten your shoulders.
- Shut your eyes and concentrate on unwinding.
- Hold for three to five minutes.

3. ***Mild Arm Stretches***
   - While sitting comfortably, lift one arm forward.
   - To extend the arm, gently push the fingers.
   - Switch arms after 30 seconds of holding.
   - Repeat each side two to three times.

Health Benefits: The Bedtime Wind-Down Poses help you unwind and get ready for a good night's sleep by calming your body and mind. These soft motions relieve stress and guarantee a calm end to the day and a sound sleep at night.

Make adjustments to these routines to suit your requirements and comfort as you incorporate them into your regular life. To fully benefit from chair yoga and achieve a harmonic balance in your physical and emotional well-being, consistency is essential.

CHAPTER 8

Customizing Yoga Positions to Meet Everybody's Needs

Yoga's versatility makes it suitable for people with different needs and capacities, which is one of its many wonderful qualities. Here's a guide on chair yoga adaptations for those with restricted mobility, how to adjust poses for varying ability levels, and answers to frequently asked issues and concerns:

Adapting Pose to Various Abilities

1. *Sitting Mountain Pose*
   - *Standard Pose:* Raise your arms high while sitting with your feet flat on the floor.
   - *Modification:* Keep your arms resting on your thighs and concentrate on activating your

core muscles if you have restricted movement.

2. ***Balance-Inducing Leg Extensions***
   - ***Standard Pose:*** Raise and straighten one leg.
   - ***Modification:*** For more assistance, use a resistance band or do smaller leg lifts.

3. ***Seated Twist for Spinal Mobility***
   - ***Standard Pose:*** Twist your torso while sitting to improve your spinal mobility.
   - ***Modification:*** If you have back problems, lessen the amount of twist or utilize a chair to provide additional support.

Principles of Adaptation

- ***Limited Range of Motion:*** Modify the range of motion to fit your comfort level.

- **_Use of Props:_** For extra support, use props like yoga blocks or cushions.
- **_Chair Support:_** When doing standing poses, use the chair to maintain balance and stability.

Chair Yoga for Those with Limited Mobility

1. **_Seated Cat-Cow Stretch_**: Take a seat, arch your back, and exhale to round your spine.
2. **_Mild Arm Stretches:_** While seated comfortably, extend one arm at a time, paying close attention to the moderate motions.
3. **_Wrist and Ankle Flexes:_** To increase joint mobility while seated, do wrist and ankle circles.

Principles of Chair Yoga for Limited Mobility

- **Seated Variations:** To improve accessibility, convert standard postures into seated variations.
- **Supportive Props:** For more comfort and support, use pillows or cushions.

Answering Frequently Asked Questions and Providing Clarity and Comfort in Yoga Practice

1. Can elderly people with arthritis benefit from chair yoga?

Answer: Definitely. Because chair yoga is mild, it's a great practice for those with arthritis because it promotes joint mobility without causing tension. Different degrees of comfort and mobility may be accommodated by adjusting the sitting postures and mindful movements.

2. What is the impact of chair yoga on back pain?

Answer: In response, chair yoga may be modified to address back discomfort by emphasizing spinal alignment and mild stretches. The technique promotes appropriate posture and gentle movements, which enhance general comfort and spinal health.

3. What happens if I get hurt and can't do a specific pose?

Answer: Adjustments are essential. It is important to let your teacher know about any limits or injuries so they can adjust the postures to suit your requirements. Chair yoga is very flexible, with several modifications available for every posture to provide a secure and productive practice.

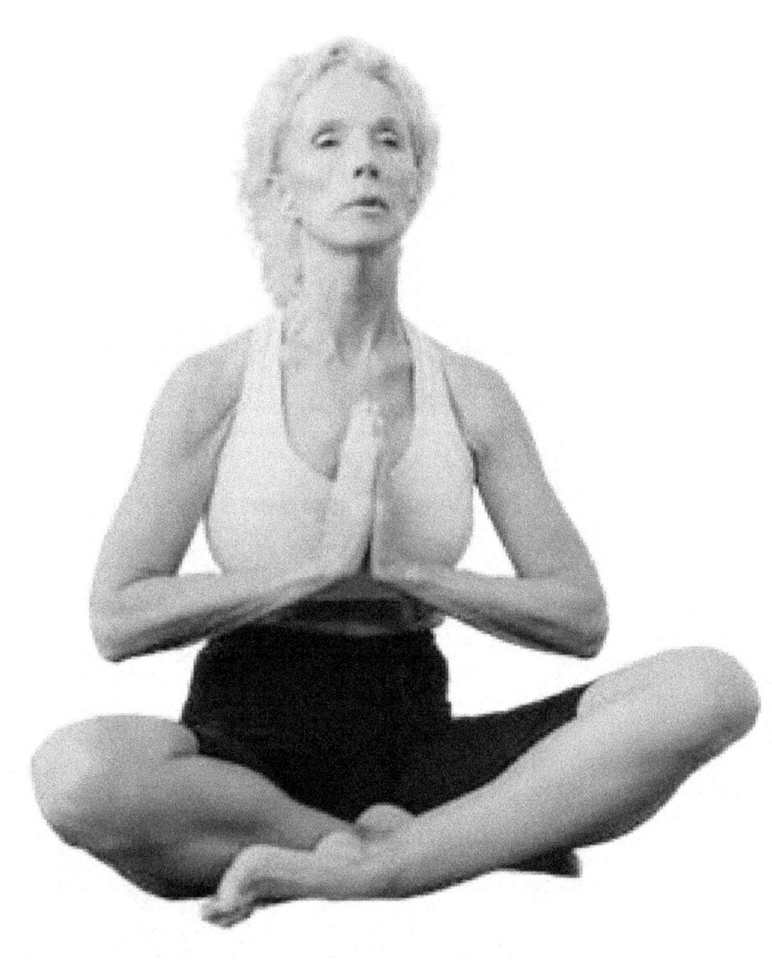

CHAPTER 9

A Holistic Approach to Wellness: Including Chair Yoga in Daily Life

Chair yoga develops into a focused, enlightening practice that enhances your general well-being and transcends beyond simple physical exercise.

1. ***Establishing a Practice Schedule That Is Regular:*** Creating a regular chair yoga practice routine is essential to integrating it into everyday life. Pick a time that fits in with your everyday schedule, whether it in the morning to kickstart the day, during a work break, or in the evening to unwind. Maintaining consistency is essential for forming a healthy habit and making chair yoga a part of your daily routine.

2. ***Including Yoga in Everyday Tasks:*** Chair yoga does not have to be limited to a certain practice period. Include mindful movements into your everyday routine to incorporate it. For instance, take deep breaths while working at your desk, stretch when seated while watching TV, or do relaxation exercises before going to bed. These short sessions help you incorporate chair yoga more deeply into your daily routine, which improves both your physical and emotional health.

3. ***Fostering Social Cohesion via Group Activities:*** Doing chair yoga with others has a social element that may be very fulfilling. Plan get-togethers with loved ones, coworkers, or friends. This encourages a feeling of community and offers encouragement and support to one another. Group yoga sessions,

whether in person or digitally, provide a supportive atmosphere where students may talk about their accomplishments, difficulties, and new perspectives, enhancing the practice in general.

<u>*Practical tips to help improve your routine*</u>

- ***Set Reminders:*** Remind yourself to do your planned chair yoga practice by setting an alarm or using calendar alerts. Establishing a habit requires consistency.
- ***Integrate Yoga with Breaks:*** Include chair yoga in your work breaks. Easy stretches and deliberate breathing are good ways to decompress and clear your head.
- ***Family Involvement:*** Invite your family to participate in your chair yoga practices. This enhances family ties and encourages a shared commitment to wellbeing.

- ***Make Use of Online Resources:*** Look into online groups and chair yoga courses. Virtual sessions provide a feeling of belonging by providing flexibility and the chance to interact with like-minded people.

- ***Honor Milestones:*** Celebrate and acknowledge your accomplishments. Acknowledging successes whether they be better posture, less stress, or more flexibility—confirms the beneficial effects of chair yoga on your day-to-day activities.

Chair yoga may be incorporated into everyday activities, practiced on a regular schedule, and group sessions can help you develop a holistic approach to wellbeing in addition to making chair yoga a regular part of your routine.

CONCLUSION

Embrace wellness through chair yoga.

Let's pause to acknowledge the many advantages that chair yoga for seniors offers as we draw to a close our investigation of this practice. Chair yoga is more than just a set of exercises; it's a comprehensive approach to health that addresses mental, emotional, and physical aspects of life.

Honoring Chair Yoga's Benefits for Seniors

We've covered the gentle stretches, conscious movements, and deep breathing that make up chair yoga on these pages. We've seen firsthand how these easily available routines improve core strength, increase flexibility, and reduce stress. Chair yoga is a life-giving practice that may help seniors feel more balanced, have less joint discomfort, and have an overall better feeling of wellbeing.

Motivation to Maintain Physical Activity and Good Health

Chair yoga is a never-ending adventure that explores the body's potential and cultivates a tranquil mind. Let us end by encouraging all seniors to continue breathing, exercising, and putting their health first. Chair yoga celebrates your body's amazing resilience, the pleasure of movement, and the embrace of a focused breath. It is not about perfection.

Recall that the chair is an instrument for empowerment, not a restriction. Your wellbeing is enhanced by all of your stretches, twists, and quiet moments. Therefore, may chair yoga be your continuous companion on your road to health and vitality, whether you're just beginning or are already well along in it.

Let the chair yoga energy continue to permeate your everyday life as we end this chapter. Appreciate the advantages you've gained, and let the inspiration to keep going resonate inside you. The practice is your road map to a rich and satisfying life, and the chair is your place of empowerment. Let's toast to the bliss of chair yoga and the unwavering will to maintain good health throughout life.

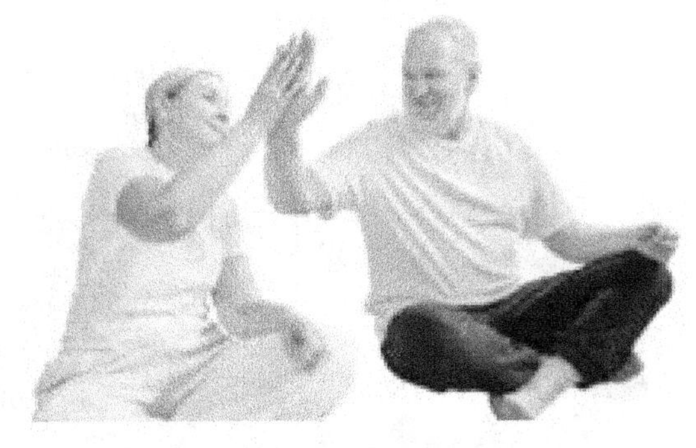

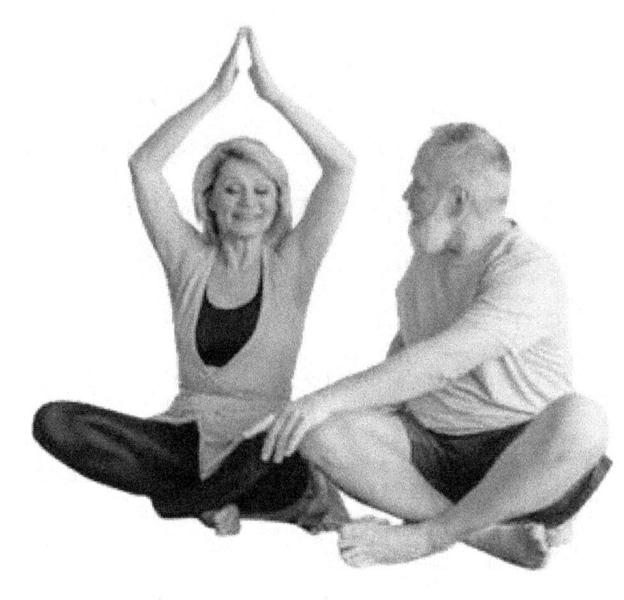

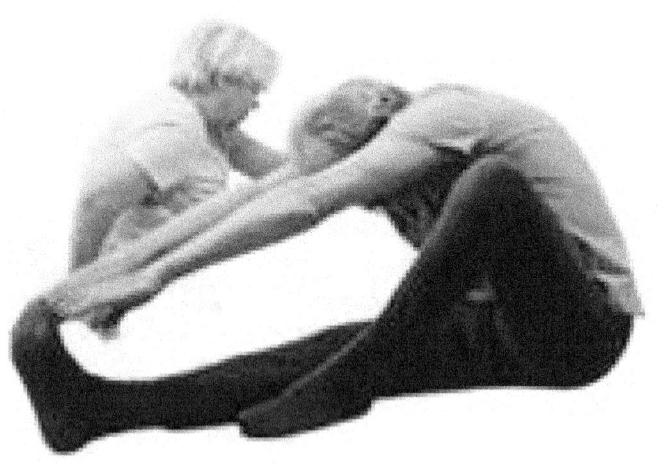

Bonus

Mental wellness through mindful moments

Welcome to the Mindful Moments bonus section, created especially to improve mental health when combined with senior chair yoga poses. Use these easy mindfulness exercises to develop a calm and peaceful attitude:

1. <u>*Guided Breathing Exercise for Relaxation*</u>

   - Take a comfortable seat with your feet flat on the ground.
   - Shut your eyes and count to four while inhaling deeply through your nose.
   - For four counts, hold your breath.
   - Take a leisurely, six-count breath out through your lips.

- Allow your breathing to become regular and slow as you repeat this cycle more times.

2. <u>*Body Scan Meditation*</u>

- Take a comfortable seat or lay down. Shut your eyes.

- Keep your focus on your toes. Observe all feelings without passing judgment. As you gradually raise your attention to each area of your body, let go of any stress.

- From your toes to your head, take a few breaths to focus on each part of your body and develop a calm awareness of it.

3. <u>*Keeping a gratitude journal*</u>

- Assign a set time each day to jot down three things for which you are thankful.

- Be thoughtful and precise. It may be anything as simple as a pleasant conversation or a beautiful day.
- Go over your entries often to help you maintain a positive outlook.

4. _Mindful Movement Integration_

- Give your whole attention to your motions, whether you're seated or standing.
- As you practice chair yoga, pay attention to how your muscles contract and release. Sense how your movement and breathing are in unison.
- Apply this conscious awareness to routine tasks like reaching for things or strolling.

5. _Sensory Awareness Exercise_

- Sit quietly for a time and pay attention to your surroundings.
- Pay attention to the noises in the surroundings, the fragrances in the air, and the textures of the items around you.
- Use all of your senses without passing judgment. Just watch and be grateful.

6. _Visualization Meditation_

- Shut your eyes and inhale deeply a few times.
- Visualize a peaceful scene in your head. Envision the minutiae - the hues, noises, and experiences.
- Let the uplifting energy from this vision fill you up, and use all of your senses.

7. _Affirmation Integration_

- Construct affirmations that are constructive and specifically linked to your chair yoga practice, such as `"I am strong and flexible."
- Say these affirmations aloud before, during, or after your sessions.
- As you internalize the empowering concepts, a feeling of empowerment comes from inside.

8. _Laughing Yoga Break_

- Practice yoga of laughing by pretending to laugh or by making fun gestures.
- Take a few deep breaths to begin, and then burst out laughing. Though it can seem strained at first, it often transforms into genuine laughing.

- To increase the happiness, tell others about the event.

9. _Mindful Eating Exercise_

- Before you eat, take a minute to enjoy the way your food looks and smells.
- Take your time chewing, enjoying every taste and feeling the textures and tastes of each mouthful.
- Set down your cutlery in between mouthful so that you may concentrate entirely on the act of eating.

10. _Gratitude Meditation_

- Locate a peaceful area and take a comfortable seat.
- Shut your eyes and list all the blessings in your life. Relationships, events, or even individual traits could be involved.

- Permit thankfulness to overflow into your thoughts and emotions. Say a quiet prayer of thanks or use soft affirmations.

If you follow these thorough directions, you'll eventually become second-nature with these mindfulness exercises that improve your physical and mental health as well as your chair yoga practice.

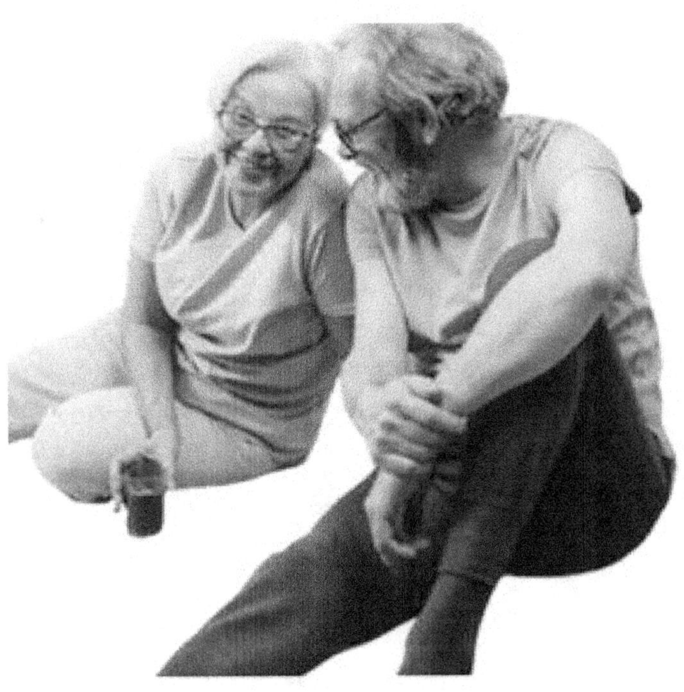

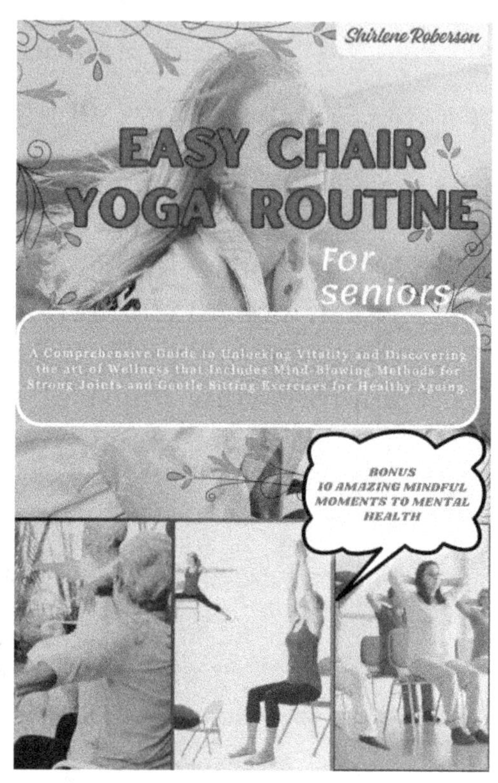

Thank You for Exploring the Path to Wellness with Our Easy Chair Yoga Routine for Seniors – Embrace Health, Embrace Life!"

www.ingramcontent.com/pod-product-compliance
Lightning Source LLC
Chambersburg PA
CBHW080942260726
48661CB00010B/4052